# The Menopause Relief

**Effective Anti-aging Tips and Hot Flash Solution: Hormones Replacement and Menopause Reset to get rid of Your Symptoms and Feel Like Your Younger Self Again**

## Patricia A. Roberson

# Table Of Contents

# Introduction

In the not-so-distant future, technology has advanced to unlock the secrets of the human body. Mary, a woman in her early 50s, faced the challenging throes of menopause. Frustration and discomfort defined her daily life until she heard of the Menopause Reset Code. It was a revolutionary breakthrough, a personalized genetic reset that promised to alleviate her symptoms and rejuvenate her like her younger self.

With a mixture of hope and trepidation, Mary chose to undergo the procedure. As the code was activated within her, a wave of transformation swept through her body. Hot flashes faded, mood swings dissolved, and her vitality returned. It wasn't just her physical health; her spirit rekindled as well.

Mary emerged from the process stronger and more vibrant than she'd been in years. The Menopause Reset Code had not only restored her youthfulness but also her zest for life. It was a testament to the power of science and determination, proving that the

challenges of aging could be met with innovation
and the courage to embrace change.

Welcome to the Menopause Reset Code, a journey
towards reclaiming your vitality, well-being, and
feeling like your younger self again. Menopause is a
natural phase of life that every woman goes through,
yet it can bring about significant physical and
emotional changes. This book is your guide to
understanding the process of menopause, its effects
on your body, and how to navigate this transitional
period with grace and confidence.

Menopause is not a destination; it's a
transformative journey. By the end of this book, you
will have the knowledge and tools to not only
manage the symptoms of menopause but also to
thrive beyond it.

**Menopause and Its Effects**
Menopause is a natural biological event that marks
the end of a woman's reproductive years. It is
defined as the cessation of menstruation for 12
consecutive months, signaling the conclusion of a
woman's fertility. While menopause is a normal
phase of life, it is often accompanied by a range of

physical, emotional, and hormonal changes that can significantly impact a woman's quality of life.

**Effects of Menopause**

Hot Flashes and Night Sweats: Hot flashes are sudden, intense feelings of heat that can spread throughout the body, often accompanied by sweating. Night sweats are hot flashes that occur during sleep, leading to disrupted sleep patterns and fatigue.

- Vaginal Dryness and Discomfort: Declining estrogen levels during menopause can lead to vaginal dryness, itching, and discomfort. These symptoms can affect sexual function and overall comfort.
- Mood Swings and Emotional Changes: Hormonal fluctuations during menopause can contribute to mood swings, irritability, anxiety, and even depression. Changes in hormone levels can affect neurotransmitters in the brain, leading to emotional instability.
- Sleep Disturbances: Menopausal women often experience sleep disturbances, including insomnia and waking up frequently

during the night. Poor sleep quality can have a cascading effect on overall well-being.

- Weight Gain and Changes in Body Composition: Many women notice changes in body composition during menopause, including an increased tendency to gain weight, particularly around the abdomen. Slower metabolism and hormonal shifts can contribute to these changes.

- Bone Health: Estrogen is essential for bone density maintenance. As estrogen levels decline during menopause, the risk of osteoporosis and fractures increases.

- Changes in Libido: Hormonal fluctuations can lead to a decrease in sexual desire and changes in sexual function. Vaginal dryness and discomfort can also impact sexual satisfaction.

- Cognitive Changes: Some women report cognitive changes during menopause, such as memory lapses and difficulty concentrating. These modifications are commonly referred to as "brain fog."

**When Does Menopause Typically Start?**

The onset of menopause varies from woman to woman, but it typically occurs between the ages of 45 and 55. However, it's important to note that menopause can occur earlier or later for some women. Menopause that occurs before the age of 40 is considered early menopause, while menopause that occurs after the age of 55 is considered late menopause.

The transition to menopause is known as perimenopause and can start several years before menopause itself. During perimenopause, hormone levels begin to fluctuate, leading to many of the symptoms associated with menopause. It's important to recognize the signs of perimenopause to better understand and manage the menopausal transition.

**Why You Can Feel Like Your Younger Self Again**

While menopause brings about a range of physical and emotional changes, it's essential to understand that it doesn't signify the end of a fulfilling and vibrant life. You can feel like your younger self again by taking proactive steps to manage and mitigate the effects of menopause.

- Hormone Replacement Therapy (HRT): Many women find relief from menopausal symptoms through hormone replacement therapy, which can help rebalance hormonal levels and alleviate hot flashes, mood swings, and other discomforts.
- Lifestyle Changes: Adopting a healthy lifestyle that includes regular exercise, a balanced diet, stress management, and adequate sleep can greatly improve your well-being during menopause.
- Herbal Remedies and Supplements: Some women turn to herbal remedies and supplements like black cohosh, soy isoflavones, and omega-3 fatty acids to alleviate menopausal symptoms.
- Mind-Body Practices: Practices such as yoga, meditation, and mindfulness can help reduce stress, improve sleep, and enhance overall mental and emotional well-being.
- Professional Support: Seeking guidance from a healthcare provider or menopause specialist can provide tailored solutions for managing menopausal symptoms and optimizing your health.

Remember, menopause is a natural phase of life, and with the right knowledge and support, you can navigate it successfully and embrace the next chapter of your life with confidence and vitality. This book is your resource for understanding, managing, and ultimately thriving during and after menopause.

# Chapter 1: The Menopause Journey

**The Menopause Journey: Navigating the Transition with Wisdom and Grace**

The menopause journey is a profound and natural phase in a woman's life that marks the end of her reproductive years. It's a transformative experience that can span several years and involves a cascade of physiological, emotional, and psychological changes. For many women, it's a time of introspection, self-discovery, and embracing a new chapter in life. Understanding the intricacies of this journey is essential for women to navigate it with wisdom and grace.

**What Is Menopause?**

Menopause, from the Greek words "meno" (month) and "pausis" (cessation), literally means "the cessation of monthly cycles." It typically occurs in women between the ages of 45 and 55, although it can happen earlier or later. Menopause signifies the end of a woman's reproductive capacity, and it's defined as the point when a woman hasn't had a menstrual period for 12 consecutive months.

However, menopause is not just a single event but a process that unfolds over several years. It involves a gradual decline in the production of key reproductive hormones, particularly estrogen and progesterone, by the ovaries. These hormonal fluctuations lead to a range of physical and emotional changes that affect each woman differently.

**Stages of Menopause**

The menopause journey is often divided into several stages, each characterized by specific hormonal, physiological, and emotional shifts. These stages provide a framework for understanding the progression of menopause and help women prepare for the changes ahead:

- Perimenopause: This is the phase leading up to menopause, usually starting in a woman's 40s but sometimes earlier. During perimenopause, hormonal fluctuations become more pronounced, leading to irregular menstrual cycles and various symptoms. It's a transitional phase that can last for several years.

- Menopause: As mentioned earlier, menopause is officially declared when a woman has not had a period for 12 consecutive months. It's a significant milestone that marks the end of fertility. Menopause usually occurs around the age of 51, but the timing varies from woman to woman.
- Postmenopause: Postmenopause refers to the years following menopause. During this stage, hormonal levels stabilize at lower levels, and many of the acute symptoms of perimenopause and early menopause begin to subside. Women are considered postmenopausal for the rest of their lives.

## Common Symptoms

The menopause journey is often accompanied by a wide range of symptoms, which can vary in intensity and duration from woman to woman. These symptoms result from hormonal fluctuations and imbalances. While not every woman will experience all of these symptoms, some of the most common ones include:

- Hot Flashes: Sudden and intense feelings of heat, often accompanied by sweating and rapid heartbeat.
- Night Sweats: Similar to hot flashes but occurring during the night, leading to disrupted sleep.
- Irregular Menstrual Cycles: Periods become unpredictable, either shorter or longer, and eventually stop altogether.
- Vaginal Dryness: Reduced estrogen levels can lead to vaginal dryness and discomfort during intercourse.
- Mood Swings: Hormonal changes can affect mood stability, leading to irritability, anxiety, or depression.
- Sleep Disturbances: Insomnia or poor-quality sleep can be common during menopause.
- Weight Gain: Changes in metabolism and hormonal imbalances may lead to weight gain, particularly around the abdomen.
- Bone Density Loss: Reduced estrogen can contribute to a decrease in bone density, increasing the risk of osteoporosis.

Understanding these common symptoms is essential for women embarking on the menopause journey. It helps them recognize the changes in their bodies, seek appropriate support and treatments, and embrace this transformative phase with resilience and self-compassion. While the menopause journey may present challenges, it can also be a time of personal growth, empowerment, and the opportunity to live life to the fullest.

# Chapter 2: Assessing Your Menopause Experience

Assessing your menopause experience is a crucial step in understanding the changes happening in your body and how they might be affecting your overall well-being. Menopause is a natural biological process, but the way it manifests can vary widely from one person to another. By taking the time to assess your menopause experience, you empower yourself to make informed decisions about your health and quality of life during this transitional phase.

One of the first aspects of assessing your menopause experience is recognizing the signs and symptoms associated with it. Menopause typically occurs between the ages of 45 and 55, with the average age being around 51. However, it can begin earlier or later for some women. The most common symptoms of menopause include hot flashes, night sweats, irregular periods, mood swings, vaginal dryness, and changes in libido. But there are many other symptoms that can be attributed to menopause as well, such as fatigue, joint pain, and memory issues.

## Recognizing Your Symptoms

Recognizing your symptoms is a fundamental part of assessing your menopause experience. It involves a deep and honest reflection on your physical, emotional, and psychological state. Here are some steps to help you recognize your symptoms effectively:

1..Self-Awareness: Start by tuning into your body and emotions. Keep a journal to record any changes or discomfort you may be experiencing. Pay attention to patterns, triggers, and the severity of symptoms. This self-awareness can be enlightening and empower you to take control of your menopause journey.

2. Educate Yourself: Learn about the common symptoms of menopause, but also be aware that your experience might differ. Knowledge is power, and understanding what you might encounter can help you recognize these symptoms when they arise.

3. Seek Help: Consult with friends, family members, or support groups. Sharing experiences and symptoms with others who are going through or have gone through menopause can provide insights and comfort. They may share coping strategies or suggest treatments that have worked for them.

4. Regular Health Check-ups: Regular check-ups with your healthcare practitioner are really important. They can help you identify symptoms you might not have recognized on your own. Routine screenings and tests can also rule out other health conditions that may mimic menopausal symptoms.

**Tracking Your Menopause Progress**
Tracking your menopause progress is a valuable tool for gaining control over this life transition. By keeping a record of your symptoms and how they evolve over time, you can identify trends, triggers, and any potential improvements. Here's how to effectively track your menopause progress:

1..Symptom Journal: Maintain a daily or weekly journal where you note your symptoms, their intensity, and any patterns you observe. Include information about your menstrual cycle, if applicable.

2. Use Apps and Tools: There are various mobile apps and online tools designed to help women track their menopause symptoms. These can provide visual representations of your progress and may even offer personalized recommendations.

3. Consult with a Specialist: Consider seeking the expertise of a menopause specialist or gynecologist. They can conduct tests to measure hormone levels, bone density, and other indicators of menopause progression. This data can provide valuable insights into your specific situation.

4. Mental and Emotional Health: Don't forget to track your mental and emotional well-being. Menopause can affect mood, anxiety levels, and overall mental health. Keeping a diary of your emotional experiences can help you address these aspects of menopause.

**Consulting with a Healthcare Professional**

Consulting with a healthcare professional is a pivotal step in your menopause journey. While self-assessment and symptom recognition are essential, a healthcare provider brings expertise and diagnostic tools to ensure you receive the appropriate care and guidance. Here's why consulting with a healthcare professional is vital during menopause:

1..Accurate Diagnosis: Menopause symptoms can overlap with those of other medical conditions. A healthcare professional can differentiate between menopause-related symptoms and other potential health issues, ensuring you receive the correct diagnosis.

2. Personalized Treatment: Your healthcare provider can tailor a treatment plan to address your specific symptoms and needs. Whether it's hormone therapy, lifestyle changes, or alternative therapies, their guidance can lead to more effective symptom management.

3. Monitoring and Safety: If you and your healthcare provider decide on hormone therapy or other medical interventions, they will monitor your

progress and assess any potential risks. Regular check-ups can ensure your treatment is safe and effective.

4. Emotional Support: Menopause can bring about emotional challenges. A healthcare professional can offer emotional support, recommend therapists or support groups, and help you navigate the psychological aspects of this life transition.

In essence, assessing your menopause experience involves recognizing your symptoms, tracking your progress, and consulting with a healthcare professional. This multifaceted approach empowers you to take control of your health during this transformative phase of life, ensuring a smoother and more informed journey through menopause. Remember, you don't have to navigate this transition alone, and seeking professional guidance is a proactive step toward better health and well-being.

# Chapter 3: The Hormonal Puzzle

The human body is a complex and finely tuned system, and at the heart of this intricate machinery lies the hormonal puzzle. Hormones are the messengers that govern many of our bodily functions, and they play a particularly prominent role in women's health, especially during the various stages of their lives. The hormonal puzzle becomes particularly fascinating and challenging during menopause, a transformative period marked by substantial shifts in hormone levels.

## Estrogen, Progesterone, and Testosterone

Three key players in this hormonal symphony are estrogen, progesterone, and testosterone. Each hormone has its unique role, and their delicate balance is essential for maintaining overall well-being.

## Estrogen:

Often referred to as the "female hormone," estrogen is primarily responsible for regulating the menstrual cycle, maintaining bone density, and supporting heart health. It plays a significant role in maintaining the elasticity and hydration of the skin, as well as in cognitive functions. As women age and approach menopause, estrogen levels begin to decline, leading to various symptoms such as hot flashes, vaginal dryness, and mood swings.

**Progesterone**:
This hormone partners with estrogen in regulating the menstrual cycle. Progesterone helps prepare the uterus for potential pregnancy by thickening the uterine lining. During menopause, progesterone production decreases, contributing to irregular periods and changes in the menstrual cycle.

**Testostcrone**:
Often associated with men, testosterone is also present in women, albeit in smaller amounts. It is essential for maintaining muscular mass, bone density, and libido. As women age, testosterone levels can decrease, leading to a decline in energy levels, muscle strength, and sexual desire.

**Hormonal Changes During Menopause**

Menopause is a natural biological process that marks the end of a woman's reproductive years. It typically occurs around the age of 45 to 55 and is characterized by a series of hormonal changes. One of the primary hormonal changes during menopause is the significant reduction in estrogen production. This decline in estrogen levels triggers a cascade of physiological alterations throughout the body.

As estrogen levels decrease, the menstrual cycle becomes irregular and eventually ceases. This transition, known as perimenopause, can bring about a wide range of symptoms, including hot flashes, night sweats, mood swings, and vaginal dryness. The hormonal fluctuations can also impact bone density, potentially increasing the risk of osteoporosis.

**How Hormones Impact Your Body**

Hormones are like conductors in an orchestra, coordinating the various instruments (organs and systems) to produce harmonious music (overall health). When hormonal balance is disrupted, it can lead to a discordant symphony of symptoms and health issues.

1..Mood and Emotions: Hormones have a strong influence on mood and emotional well-being. Fluctuations in estrogen and progesterone can contribute to mood swings, irritability, and even depression during menopause.

2. Physical Health: Estrogen plays a vital role in maintaining cardiovascular health by regulating cholesterol levels and promoting healthy blood vessel function. As estrogen levels drop, women may become more susceptible to heart disease.

3. Bone Health: Estrogen is necessary for bone density maintenance. Its decline during menopause can increase the risk of osteoporosis, a condition characterized by brittle and fragile bones.

4. Reproductive Health: Hormonal changes during menopause mark the end of a woman's reproductive capacity. The cessation of menstruation and a decrease in fertility are among the most prominent effects on reproductive health.

5. Sexual Health: Hormonal changes can also impact sexual health. Vaginal dryness and a decrease in

libido are common symptoms of declining estrogen levels.

In essence, hormones are the invisible architects of our bodies, orchestrating a symphony of functions that influence our physical, emotional, and mental well-being. Understanding the hormonal puzzle, particularly during menopause, is the first step toward managing its challenges and unlocking the potential for women to feel like their younger selves again. Hormone replacement therapy (HRT), lifestyle changes, and personalized wellness strategies are some of the tools available to navigate this intricate journey with grace and vitality.

# Chapter 4. Nutrition and Menopause

**Nutrition and Menopause: Hormone-Friendly Foods for Menopause**

Menopause is a natural and inevitable stage in a woman's life, typically occurring between the ages of 45 and 55. It marks the end of a woman's reproductive years and is accompanied by a series of hormonal changes that can result in a variety of physical and emotional symptoms. While menopause is a natural process, it can be a challenging time for many women, as it brings about symptoms such as hot flashes, night sweats, mood swings, and weight gain. Fortunately, one powerful tool in managing these symptoms is proper nutrition, and incorporating hormone-friendly foods into your diet can make a significant difference in how you experience menopause.

Hormone-friendly foods are those that support hormonal balance and overall well-being during menopause. They can help alleviate some of the discomfort associated with this life stage and promote a healthier transition. Here, we'll explore a range of hormone-friendly foods that can become valuable additions to your daily diet:

1. Phytoestrogen-Rich Foods:
   - Soy Products: Soybeans, tofu, tempeh, and soy milk contain phytoestrogens, which are plant compounds that mimic the effects of estrogen in the body. These can help alleviate hot flashes and other estrogen-related symptoms.
   - Flaxseeds: Flaxseeds are another excellent source of phytoestrogens, specifically lignans. Ground flaxseeds can be sprinkled on cereal or yogurt for an easy addition to your meals.

2. Calcium-Rich Foods:
   - Dairy Products: Low-fat dairy items like yogurt, milk, and cheese are not only rich in calcium but also provide vitamin D for better calcium absorption. This combination

supports bone health, which can be compromised during menopause.

- Leafy Greens: Broccoli, kale, collard greens, and spinach are high in calcium and other essential nutrients. Incorporating these vegetables into your diet can contribute to strong bones.

3. Omega-3 Fatty Acids:
- Fatty Fish: Salmon, mackerel, sardines, and trout are loaded with omega-3 fatty acids, which have anti-inflammatory properties and may help reduce the risk of heart disease, a concern that becomes more relevant after menopause.
- Chia Seeds and Walnuts: These plant-based sources of omega-3s can be included in salads, smoothies, or as a topping for oatmeal.

4. Fiber-Rich Foods:
- Whole Grains: Opt for whole grains like oats, quinoa, brown rice, and whole wheat bread to support digestive health and regulate blood sugar levels.

- Fruits and Vegetables: A colorful variety of fruits and vegetables provides essential fiber, vitamins, and minerals. Fiber helps with digestion and can assist in weight management.

5. Lean Protein Sources:
   - Lean Meats: Skinless poultry, lean cuts of beef, and pork are excellent sources of protein without excessive saturated fats.
   - Legumes: Beans, lentils, and chickpeas are rich in protein, fiber, and various essential nutrients. They can be included in soups, salads, and stews.

6. Fruits and Berries:

Berries, such as blueberries, strawberries, and raspberries, are high in antioxidants, which combat oxidative stress and inflammation. They're also low in calories and can satisfy sweet cravings in a healthy way.

6. Water and Hydration:

Staying well-hydrated is crucial during menopause, as it can help alleviate symptoms like hot flashes and night sweats. Drink plenty of water throughout the day, and consider herbal teas for added hydration and relaxation.

Incorporating these hormone-friendly foods into your diet can help you manage the hormonal fluctuations and symptoms that often accompany menopause. It's essential to consult with a healthcare professional or nutritionist to create a personalized nutrition plan tailored to your specific needs and preferences. Additionally, adopting a well-balanced diet, along with regular exercise and stress management, can significantly enhance your overall quality of life during this transformative phase. Remember that proper nutrition is a key component of a holistic approach to managing menopause and promoting long-term well-being.

**Foods to Avoid During Menopause:**
Processed and Sugary Foods: Highly processed foods, sugary snacks, and sugary beverages can lead to weight gain and worsen mood swings and hot flashes. They can also disrupt blood sugar levels.

- Caffeine and Alcohol: Both caffeine and alcohol can interfere with sleep patterns, which are already disrupted in many menopausal women. Limit your intake, especially in the evening, to improve sleep quality.

- Spicy Foods: Spicy meals might cause or aggravate hot flashes and nocturnal sweats in certain women. If you notice this effect, reduce your consumption of spicy dishes.
- High-Sodium Foods: Excess sodium can contribute to bloating and water retention, which may be more noticeable during menopause. Reduce your intake of salty snacks and processed foods.
- Red Meat: High consumption of red meat has been linked to an increased risk of heart disease and may exacerbate some menopausal symptoms. Choose lean cuts of meat and consider plant-based protein sources more often.
- Fried Foods: Fried foods are high in harmful fats and might contribute to weight gain. They can also lead to digestive discomfort, which may already be a concern during menopause.
- Excessive Dairy: While dairy is important for calcium intake, consuming too much full-fat

dairy can lead to weight gain. Opt for low-fat or dairy alternatives when possible.

It's essential to remember that individual responses to specific foods can vary, so it's a good idea to keep a food journal and pay attention to how different foods affect your symptoms. Consulting with a registered dietitian or healthcare provider can also provide personalized guidance on dietary choices during menopause, ensuring you're making the best choices for your unique needs and preferences.

## Meal Planning

Meal planning for menopause is a crucial aspect of managing the physical and emotional changes that women experience during this life stage. Menopause is a natural biological process that marks the end of a woman's reproductive years, typically occurring between the ages of 45 and 55. During this time, hormonal fluctuations, particularly a decrease in estrogen, can lead to a range of symptoms, including hot flashes, night sweats, mood swings, weight gain, and changes in metabolism. A well-balanced and thoughtfully designed meal plan can help alleviate some of these symptoms, support overall health, and contribute to a smoother transition through menopause.

1. Balancing Hormones:
Hormonal imbalances are at the core of many menopausal symptoms. Estrogen, progesterone, and testosterone levels can fluctuate significantly, affecting mood, energy levels, and weight management. Meal planning for menopause should prioritize foods that promote hormonal balance. This includes:

- Phytoestrogens: Foods rich in phytoestrogens, such as soy products, flaxseeds, and legumes, can help mimic the effects of estrogen in the body and alleviate some symptoms.
- Healthy Fats: Omega-3 fatty acids found in fatty fish like salmon, as well as in walnuts and chia seeds, can help regulate hormone production.
- Protein: Adequate protein intake is essential for maintaining muscle mass, which can decrease during menopause due to hormonal

changes. Lean sources of protein like poultry, tofu, and beans are excellent choices.

2. Supporting Bone Health:
Menopause is a time when women are at an increased risk of developing osteoporosis due to a drop in estrogen levels. A meal plan for menopause should include foods rich in calcium and vitamin D, which are essential for maintaining strong bones. Dairy products, leafy greens, fortified foods, and supplements when necessary, can help protect bone health.

3. Managing Weight:
Many women notice changes in body composition during menopause, including an increase in abdominal fat. Proper meal planning can assist in managing weight and preventing excess fat gain. Key strategies include:

- Portion Control: Paying attention to portion sizes to avoid overeating.

- Balanced Meals: Prioritizing lean proteins, whole grains, and plenty of vegetables to create satisfying and nutrient-dense meals.
- Fiber: High-fiber foods like whole grains, fruits, and vegetables can help with appetite control and digestion.

4. Reducing Hot Flashes and Night Sweats:

Certain foods and beverages can trigger hot flashes and night sweats in some women. It's essential to identify these triggers and avoid them in your meal plan. Spicy foods, coffee, alcohol, and hot beverages are all common triggers.

5. Mood and Cognitive Health:

Menopause can also affect mood and cognitive function. Nutrient-rich foods can support brain health and emotional well-being. Foods high in antioxidants, such as berries, leafy greens, and nuts, can protect brain cells and enhance mood stability.

6. Hydration:

Staying well-hydrated is crucial during menopause. Hormonal changes can lead to dry skin and mucous membranes, so it's important to drink enough water throughout the day. Herbal teas, like chamomile and peppermint, can also be soothing and hydrating.

7. Consulting a Healthcare Professional:

It's essential to tailor your meal plan to your individual needs. Consulting with a healthcare professional, such as a registered dietitian, can help you create a personalized meal plan that addresses your specific symptoms and dietary preferences.

## Supplements and Nutritional Support: Enhancing Wellness During Menopause

As women age and go through menopause, their bodies undergo significant changes. The hormonal fluctuations can lead to symptoms such as hot flashes, night sweats, mood swings, and changes in metabolism. Additionally, menopause can have long-term effects on bone density and cardiovascular health. Supplements and nutritional support can play a crucial role in mitigating these challenges.

## Key Nutrients for Menopausal Women

- Calcium and Vitamin D: Maintaining strong bones is a paramount concern for menopausal women, as hormonal changes can lead to bone density loss. Calcium and vitamin D supplements can help fortify bones and reduce the risk of fractures.

- Omega-3 Fatty Acids: Omega-3s, found in fatty fish and flaxseeds, have anti-inflammatory properties and can support heart health. Many menopausal women experience changes in cholesterol levels and blood pressure, making omega-3 supplementation beneficial.
- Magnesium: Magnesium is vital for muscle and nerve function, and it may help alleviate symptoms like muscle cramps and insomnia that some women experience during menopause.
- B Vitamins: B vitamins, including B6 and B12, are essential for mood regulation and cognitive function. Menopausal women often struggle with mood swings and cognitive changes, making these vitamins valuable.
- Iron: While women generally require less iron after menopause, some may still need supplementation if they have heavy menstrual bleeding or a deficiency.
- Phytoestrogens: Certain plant compounds, such as isoflavones found in soy, may help mitigate some menopausal symptoms by

acting as weak estrogens in the body. These can be consumed through supplements or dietary sources.

## Herbal Remedies and Botanical Supplements

In addition to essential nutrients, menopausal women often explore herbal remedies and botanical supplements for symptom relief. Some popular options include:

- Black Cohosh: Widely studied for its potential to reduce hot flashes and mood swings.
- Red Clover: Contains isoflavones and may help alleviate hot flashes and night sweats.
- Dong Quai: A traditional Chinese herb believed to support hormonal balance.
- Evening Primrose Oil: Contains gamma-linolenic acid (GLA) and may help with breast pain and mood swings.
- Chasteberry (Vitex): May help regulate hormone levels and alleviate menstrual irregularities.

It's important to note that herbal supplements can interact with medications and have varying degrees of effectiveness for different individuals. Consulting with a healthcare provider before adding herbal remedies to your regimen is advisable.

## Safety and Quality Assurance

When considering supplements during menopause, it's crucial to prioritize safety and quality. The dietary supplement industry is vast, and not all products are created equal. Look for supplements that have been independently tested for purity and potency by organizations like the United States Pharmacopeia (USP) or NSF International.

Furthermore, before beginning any new supplement regimen, always consult with a healthcare practitioner. They can assess your specific needs, potential interactions with medications, and any underlying health conditions that might affect your supplement choices.

## The Holistic Approach

Supplements and nutritional support are just one facet of managing menopause symptoms. An integrative approach that includes a balanced diet, regular exercise, stress management, and good sleep hygiene is essential for overall well-being during this life stage. Additionally, discussing your supplement choices with a healthcare provider as part of a comprehensive menopause management plan can help ensure that you are taking the most suitable and effective steps toward optimizing your health and comfort during menopause.

# Chapter 5: Exercise for Hormonal Balance

**Exercise for Hormonal Balance: The Key to Menopausal Well-being**

Menopause is a transformative phase in a woman's life, marked by fluctuating hormone levels and a myriad of physical and emotional changes. During this time, the body undergoes a significant hormonal shift, particularly in the levels of estrogen, progesterone, and testosterone. These hormonal fluctuations can lead to symptoms like hot flashes, mood swings, weight gain, and a decrease in bone density. However, the good news is that incorporating exercise into your daily routine can play a pivotal role in restoring hormonal balance and alleviating many of these symptoms.

## The Importance of Physical Activity

Physical activity is the cornerstone of a healthy lifestyle at any age, and it becomes even more crucial during menopause. Exercise offers a wide range of benefits, both for your physical and emotional well-being and can be a powerful tool for managing the hormonal changes that accompany menopause.

1..Weight Management: Menopause often brings about an increased tendency to gain weight, especially around the abdomen. Regular exercise helps to control weight by boosting metabolism and burning calories. It also helps maintain lean muscle mass, which can decline with age.

2. Hormonal Regulation: Exercise influences the release of various hormones, including endorphins (the body's natural mood lifters) and insulin (which helps regulate blood sugar levels). Engaging in physical activity can help stabilize hormonal fluctuations, leading to improved mood and energy levels.

3. Bone Health: Osteoporosis, a condition characterized by weakened bones, is a concern for many women during and after menopause due to declining estrogen levels. Weight-bearing exercises, such as walking and strength training, can help increase bone density and reduce the risk of fractures.

4. Cardiovascular Health: Menopause is associated with an increased risk of heart disease. Aerobic exercises like brisk walking, jogging, or swimming can strengthen the heart, lower blood pressure, and improve circulation.

5. Stress Reduction: The menopausal transition can bring about significant stress and anxiety. Regular physical activity acts as a natural stress reliever, promoting relaxation and mental clarity.

**Tailoring Your Exercise Routine**

Creating an exercise routine that suits your needs and preferences is essential for long-term adherence and effectiveness. Here are some key considerations when tailoring your exercise routine during menopause:

1..Assess Your Current Fitness Level: Before starting any exercise program, it's essential to evaluate your current fitness level. This evaluation will assist you in determining your starting place and setting reasonable goals.

2. Choose Activities You Enjoy: The most effective exercise routine is one you'll stick to. Select activities that you genuinely enjoy, whether it's dancing, hiking, swimming, or playing a sport. Adding variety to your routines can also keep them interesting and prevent monotony.

3. Set Realistic Goals: Establish achievable fitness goals that align with your menopause-related concerns. For instance, if your primary concern is bone health, prioritize weight-bearing exercises. If you're focused on stress reduction, incorporate relaxation practices like yoga and Pilates.

4. Create a Balanced Routine: Aim for a mix of aerobic, strength-training, flexibility, and balance exercises. A balanced routine ensures you address various aspects of health and fitness.

## Yoga, Pilates, and Mind-Body Practices

Yoga, Pilates, and mind-body practices are exceptional choices for women going through menopause. These activities not only offer physical benefits but also promote mental well-being and mindfulness.

**Yoga**: Yoga is a complete practice that incorporates physical postures, breathing exercises, and meditation. It enhances flexibility, balance, and strength while reducing stress and promoting relaxation. Specific yoga poses, such as the "bridge pose" or "cobra pose," can target areas affected by menopausal symptoms.

**Pilates**: Pilates focuses on core strength, stability, and flexibility. It can help alleviate lower back pain, a common complaint during menopause. Pilates exercises are often performed on a mat or specialized equipment and are adaptable to different fitness levels.

**Mind-Body Practices:** Mindfulness meditation, tai chi, and qigong are mind-body practices that can be highly beneficial for managing stress, improving mood, and enhancing overall well-being. These practices emphasize the mind-body connection and can be integrated into your exercise routine.

Incorporating exercise for hormonal balance into your daily life can be a game-changer during menopause. It not only helps mitigate the physical and emotional challenges but also empowers you to embrace this new phase of life with vitality and confidence. Remember that consulting with a healthcare professional or fitness expert can provide personalized guidance tailored to your unique needs and circumstances.

As women transition through menopause, they often seek exercise routines that not only help manage physical symptoms but also promote mental and emotional well-being. Pilates, yoga, and mind-body practices are popular choices due to their holistic approach to fitness, offering a range of benefits that can be particularly valuable during this life stage

**Types of Pilates Exercises:**

Mat Pilates: Mat Pilates is a fundamental form of Pilates that can be practiced anywhere, using only a mat or a soft surface. Here are some key exercises:

1..The Hundred: Lie on your back with your knees bent, lift your head and shoulders, and pump your arms vigorously while breathing in for five counts and out for five counts.

2. The Roll-Up: Begin lying on your back with your legs straight. Roll up to a sitting position, reach forward, and then roll back down to the mat with control.

3. The Plank: Start in a push-up position but with your forearms on the ground. Maintain a straight line with your body and engage your core.

4. Reformer Pilates: Reformer exercises are performed on a specialized machine equipped with springs, straps, and a moving carriage. Some common exercises include:

- Leg Circles: Lie on your back with your legs extended on the carriage. Circle one leg while keeping the other still, then reverse the direction.
- Short Box Series: Sit on the box (a cushioned apparatus) and perform exercises that target the core and upper body, such as the twist, side lift, and back extension.

5. Cadillac (Trap Table) Pilates: The Cadillac is a versatile piece of Pilates equipment with various attachments, including bars, straps, and springs. Exercises include:

- Leg Springs: Attach leg springs to your ankles and perform exercises like leg lifts and circles.
- Roll-Down Bar: Lie on your back, hold the roll-down bar, and articulate your spine as you roll up and down.

6. Wunda Chair Pilates: The Wunda Chair is a compact piece of equipment used for seated and standing exercises. Examples include:

- Chair Squats: Sit on the chair with your feet on the pedal. Press the pedal down while standing and then return to the seated position.
- Horseback: Sit on the chair facing backward, grip the handles, and press the pedal down while maintaining an upright posture.

**Types of Yoga Exercises and How to Practice Them**:

**1..Hatha Yoga**: Hatha is a gentle and foundational style of yoga, perfect for beginners. It emphasizes physical postures and alignment. To practice Hatha yoga:

- Start with basic poses like Mountain Pose (Tadasana), Downward Dog (Adho Mukha Svanasana), and Child's Pose (Balasana).
- Focus on breath awareness and holding poses for several breaths.

**2. Vinyasa Yoga:** Vinyasa is a dynamic, flowing style of yoga that synchronizes breath with movement. To practice Vinyasa yoga:
- Warm up with Sun Salutations (Surya Namaskar).
- Flow through a sequence of poses, linking each movement with a breath.

**3. Ashtanga Yoga**: Ashtanga is a rigorous, structured style of yoga that follows a specific sequence of postures. To practice Ashtanga yoga:
- Learn the Primary Series and progress through it as you become more proficient.
- Focus on deep, even breaths and maintaining a strong, engaged core.

**4. Bikram Yoga**: Bikram yoga consists of a series of 26 postures practiced in a room heated to a high temperature. To practice Bikram yoga:

- Prepare to sweat profusely and stay hydrated.
- Follow the instructor's cues through each posture in the sequence.

**5. Iyengar Yoga:** Iyengar is a precise and alignment-focused style of yoga that often uses props like blocks and belts. To practice Iyengar yoga:

- Pay close attention to alignment and use props to support your practice.
- Hold poses for an extended period to deepen the stretch and enhance alignment.

## Mind-Body Practices: Nurturing Mental and Emotional Well-being

Mind-body practices encompass a variety of techniques that promote harmony between the mind, body, and spirit. These practices can reduce stress, enhance self-awareness, and improve mental well-being. Here, we'll explore some common mind-body practices and how to incorporate them into your routine.

**Types of Mind-Body Practices:**

**1.Meditation:** Meditation entails focusing your attention and removing the stream of thoughts that may be clogging your head. To meditate, do the following:

- Locate a quiet and pleasant location.
- Close your eyes and take deep, slow breaths while sitting or lying down.
- Pay attention to your breathing, a mantra, or a guided meditation.

**2. Breathwork:** Breathwork techniques involve conscious control of the breath to influence mental and emotional states. To practice breathwork:

- Choose a specific technique, such as deep diaphragmatic breathing or alternate nostril breathing.
- Practice regularly to reduce stress and increase relaxation.

**3. Progressive Muscle Relaxation:** This technique involves systematically tensing and relaxing muscle groups to release physical tension and promote relaxation. To practice progressive muscle relaxation:

- Begin at the toes and work your way up, tensing and then relaxing each muscle group.
- Focus on the sensation of relaxation as you release tension in each muscle.

Mind-body practices can be integrated into your daily routine to enhance your mental and emotional well-being. Whether you choose yoga, Pilates, meditation, or other techniques, these practices offer valuable tools for managing stress, improving self-awareness, and promoting a sense of inner balance and harmony.

# Chapter 6:Stress Management and Sleep

Stress and sleep are interconnected aspects of our lives, with the potential to greatly influence our overall well-being. In the context of menopause, managing stress and improving sleep quality becomes paramount for women navigating this transformative phase. Let's delve extensively into how stress impacts menopause, explore techniques for stress reduction, and discuss strategies for enhancing sleep during this critical time.

## Stress's Impact on Menopause

Menopause is a physiological process that marks the end of a woman's reproductive years. It typically occurs in the late 40s or early 50s and involves a significant shift in hormonal balance, primarily a decrease in estrogen and progesterone production. This hormonal upheaval can lead to a range of physical and emotional symptoms, including hot flashes, mood swings, anxiety, and sleep disturbances. Stress, both chronic and acute, can exacerbate these symptoms.

The relationship between stress and menopause is bidirectional. Menopause itself can be a stressful experience due to the physical discomfort and emotional changes it brings. Conversely, stress can worsen menopausal symptoms, making the transition more challenging. Stress triggers the release of cortisol, the body's primary stress hormone. Elevated cortisol levels can disrupt the already delicate hormonal balance, intensifying symptoms like hot flashes, mood swings, and insomnia.

## Techniques for Stress Reduction

Effective stress management techniques are vital for women going through menopause. Reducing stress not only alleviates the severity of menopausal symptoms but also promotes overall well-being.

Here are some techniques to consider:
1..Mindfulness Meditation: Mindfulness practices teach you to stay present and non-judgmentally aware of your thoughts and feelings. This can help reduce stress by promoting relaxation and emotional balance.

2. Deep Breathing Exercises: Deep, diaphragmatic breathing can activate the body's relaxation response, counteracting the stress-induced fight-or-flight response. Techniques like belly breathing can be practiced daily to manage stress.

3. Yoga and Tai Chi: These mind-body practices combine gentle physical movements with breath control and meditation. They promote relaxation, reduce muscle tension, and enhance overall well-being.

4. Regular Exercise: Exercise on a regular basis releases endorphins, which are the body's natural stress relievers. It also helps with weight management and overall health.

5. Counseling or Therapy: Talking to a therapist or counselor can provide a safe space to address the emotional challenges of menopause and develop coping strategies.

6. Time Management and Prioritization: Simplifying your schedule, setting realistic goals, and learning to

say no when necessary can reduce the stress associated with feeling overwhelmed.

**Improving Sleep Quality**

Sleep disturbances are common during menopause, but they are not insurmountable. Improving sleep quality is crucial for managing menopausal symptoms and ensuring overall health and vitality.

Here are strategies for enhancing sleep:
1..Create a Relaxing Bedtime Routine: Establish calming rituals before bedtime, such as reading, gentle stretching, or taking a warm bath. This signals to your body that it's time to wind down.

2. Keep a Consistent Sleep Schedule: Go to bed and wake up at the same times every day, even on weekends. Consistency reinforces your body's natural sleep-wake cycle.

3. Limit Stimulants and Screen Time: Avoid caffeine and electronic devices with blue light in the hours leading up to bedtime. These can make it difficult to fall asleep.

4. Optimize Your Sleep Environment: Make your bedroom a sanctuary for sleep by keeping it dark, cool, and quiet. Always use a comfortable mattress and pillows.

5. Mindful Nutrition: Avoid heavy meals and alcohol close to bedtime, as they can disrupt sleep. Consider a light, balanced snack if you're hungry before bed.

6. Manage Stress: Implement stress-reduction techniques (as discussed earlier) to calm your mind and reduce anxiety that can keep you awake at night.

7. Consider Hormone Therapy: In consultation with a healthcare provider, hormone therapy may be an option for some women to alleviate severe menopausal symptoms, including sleep disturbances.

# Chapter 7: Herbal Remedies and Supplements

Herbal remedies and supplements have gained significant popularity as a natural approach to managing menopausal symptoms. Many women seek alternatives to hormone replacement therapy (HRT) and pharmaceuticals, turning to herbs and supplements for relief. These natural options offer a holistic approach to addressing the physical and emotional changes that often accompany menopause.

## Herbal Options for Menopause

Black Cohosh: One of the most well-known herbal remedies for menopause, black cohosh, is derived from the root of the plant. It is believed to help alleviate hot flashes, night sweats, and mood swings. While research on its effectiveness is ongoing, some women report significant relief from their symptoms after using black cohosh.

- Red Clover: This herb contains compounds called isoflavones, which are similar to phytoestrogens. Red clover may help reduce hot flashes and improve bone health. However, the consequences differ from person to person.
- Dong Quai: Often referred to as the "female ginseng," dong quai is used in traditional Chinese medicine to address menopausal symptoms such as hot flashes and vaginal dryness. It may also support overall reproductive health.
- Soy Isoflavones: Soy products are rich in isoflavones, which mimic estrogen in the body. Some women find relief from hot flashes and mood swings by increasing their soy intake. This approach is especially popular among vegetarians and vegans.
- Evening Primrose Oil: This oil is a source of gamma-linolenic acid (GLA), an essential fatty acid. It may help alleviate breast tenderness, mood swings, and dry skin during menopause.

- Chasteberry (Vitex): Chasteberry is known for its potential to regulate hormonal imbalances, making it useful for managing symptoms like irregular periods and mood swings.
- Ginseng: Ginseng is an adaptogenic herb that may help reduce fatigue and boost energy levels, which can be beneficial for women experiencing menopausal exhaustion.

It's essential to consult with a healthcare professional before incorporating herbal remedies into your menopause management plan. What works for one woman may not work for another, and it's crucial to consider potential interactions with medications or existing health conditions.

## Vitamin and Mineral Supplements

Vitamins and minerals play a vital role in overall health, and their importance doesn't diminish during menopause. In fact, some nutrients become even more critical during this life stage:

- Calcium: Adequate calcium intake is crucial for maintaining bone health, as menopause is associated with a decline in bone density.

Women should consider calcium supplements or calcium-rich foods like dairy products, fortified non-dairy milk, and leafy greens.

- Vitamin D: Vitamin D helps the body absorb calcium and is essential for bone health. It also plays a role in mood regulation. Many women may benefit from vitamin D supplements, particularly if they have limited sun exposure.
- Magnesium: This mineral supports muscle function, and relaxation, and may help reduce menopausal symptoms like muscle cramps and mood swings.
- B Vitamins: B vitamins, especially B6, B12, and folic acid, are essential for mood regulation and overall energy levels. These vitamins can be obtained through a balanced diet or supplements.
- Omega-3 Fatty Acids: Omega-3 supplements, often sourced from fish oil, may help reduce inflammation and alleviate mood swings and joint discomfort.

## Safety and Effectiveness

While herbal remedies and supplements offer potential benefits for menopausal symptom relief, it's crucial to approach them with caution:

- Safety: Not all herbal remedies are safe for everyone. Some may interfere with drugs or worsen existing medical issues. Before beginning any new supplement, always with your doctor.
- Effectiveness: The effectiveness of herbal medicines and supplements varies greatly from person to person. What works for one woman might not work for the next. It is critical to have realistic expectations and to be patient while experimenting with various choices.
- Quality Matters: When purchasing supplements, choose reputed brands and products. To assure purity and potency, look for third-party testing and quality certificates.
- Potential Side Effects: Some herbal medicines and supplements may induce negative effects such as gastrointestinal distress or allergic responses. Monitor your

body's reaction and stop using if any negative
effects develop.

# Chapter 8: Bioidentical Hormone Replacement Therapy (BHRT)

**Bioidentical Hormone Replacement Therapy (BHRT): Unlocking the Potential of Natural Hormones**

Bioidentical Hormone Replacement Therapy (BHRT) is a therapeutic approach gaining popularity among menopausal and postmenopausal women, as well as men experiencing hormone imbalances. BHRT is distinct from conventional hormone replacement therapy (HRT) due to its use of hormones that are molecularly identical to those naturally produced by the human body. In this in-depth exploration of BHRT, we delve into its intricacies, risks, benefits, and the crucial conversation one should have with a healthcare provider before embarking on this journey to hormonal balance.

**Understanding BHRT**

BHRT is rooted in the concept of bioidentical hormones, which are chemically indistinguishable from the hormones the human body generates. These hormones, typically estrogen, progesterone, and testosterone, play vital roles in regulating various bodily functions, including metabolism, mood, and reproductive health. As individuals age, hormone levels may fluctuate and decline, resulting in symptoms like hot flashes, mood swings, and reduced libido.

BHRT seeks to restore hormonal balance by replacing deficient hormones with bioidentical counterparts. Unlike synthetic hormones used in traditional HRT, bioidentical hormones are derived from natural sources, such as yams or soy, and then modified to match human hormones precisely. This customization minimizes the risk of adverse effects associated with synthetic hormones.

**Risks and Benefits**

Before considering BHRT, it is crucial to assess both its potential advantages and risks.

**Benefits of BHRT:**

- Symptom Relief: BHRT is known for its efficacy in alleviating menopausal symptoms like hot flashes, night sweats, and mood swings.
- Hormonal Balance: BHRT aims to restore hormonal balance, which can contribute to improved overall well-being, including better sleep, mental clarity, and energy levels.
- Bone Health: BHRT may help maintain bone density and reduce the risk of osteoporosis, a common concern for postmenopausal women.
- Heart Health: Some studies suggest that BHRT may have a positive impact on cardiovascular health by improving lipid profiles and reducing the risk of heart disease.

**Risks of BHRT:**

- Side Effects: Although BHRT uses bioidentical hormones, there can still be side effects, such as breast tenderness, mood swings, and headaches, especially if the dosing is incorrect.
- 

- Lack of Long-term Research: Long-term studies on BHRT are limited, making it challenging to fully assess its safety and potential risks.
- Individual Variation: BHRT isn't one-size-fits-all. The effectiveness and tolerance of BHRT can vary from person to person, and finding the right balance may require time and adjustments.

## Discussing BHRT with Your Doctor

Engaging in an open and informed dialogue with a healthcare provider is pivotal when contemplating BHRT. Here are essential aspects to consider when discussing BHRT with your doctor:

- Medical History: Provide your doctor with a comprehensive medical history, including any pre-existing conditions, medications, and allergies, as these factors can influence the appropriateness of BHRT.
- Symptom Assessment: Clearly communicate your menopausal symptoms and their impact on your daily life. This information will help your doctor tailor BHRT to your specific needs.

- Treatment Goals: Define your treatment objectives. Are you primarily seeking symptom relief, or are you interested in long-term health benefits, such as bone preservation or cardiovascular protection?
- Risk-Benefit Analysis: Engage in a thorough discussion about the potential risks and benefits of BHRT, considering your individual health profile and concerns.
- Treatment Plan: Collaborate with your healthcare provider to establish a personalized treatment plan, including hormone type, dosage, and administration method (oral, transdermal, or pellet).
- Monitoring: Regular follow-up appointments are crucial to monitor your progress, make necessary adjustments, and ensure your safety while undergoing BHRT.

In conclusion, BHRT offers a promising path for individuals seeking relief from menopausal symptoms and hormonal imbalances. However, the decision to pursue BHRT should be made in consultation with a knowledgeable healthcare provider who can guide you through the process, ensuring that the potential benefits align with your health goals while minimizing the associated risks. BHRT, when used judiciously and monitored closely, can empower individuals to regain hormonal equilibrium and lead a healthier, more vibrant life.

# Chapter 9: Designing Your Menopause Reset

Designing your menopause reset is a crucial step in reclaiming control over your well-being during this significant life transition. Menopause is not a one-size-fits-all experience, and designing a personalized plan that aligns with your unique needs and goals is essential for a successful reset.

To begin, take some time to reflect on your current menopausal experience. What are the most bothersome symptoms you're facing? Are there specific aspects of your life, such as your energy levels, mood, or physical health, that you want to improve? Identifying your pain points and areas where you'd like to see positive changes will serve as the foundation for setting clear goals.

## Setting Clear Goals

Setting clear and specific goals is a fundamental part of your menopause reset journey. These goals will provide you with direction, motivation, and a sense of purpose as you work towards alleviating symptoms and regaining your vitality. When establishing your goals, remember the SMART criteria:

- Specific: Make your goals as precise as possible. Instead of a vague goal like "feeling better," aim for something like "reducing hot flashes by 50% in the next three months."
- Measurable: Your objectives should be quantifiable so that you can monitor your progress. To measure success, use numbers or other measurable criteria.
- Achievable: Make sure your goals are practical and feasible given your existing situation. Set realistic goals rather than overly ambitious ones that may lead to frustration.
- Relevant: Your goals should be relevant to your menopause experience and overall well-being. They should address the specific symptoms or challenges you're facing.
- 

- Time-Bound: Set a firm deadline for attaining your objectives. This creates a sense of urgency and keeps you on track. As an example, "improving sleep quality within two months."

Once you've defined your SMART goals, write them down and keep them visible. Share your goals with a trusted friend or family member to solidify your commitment and gain their support.

## Creating a Menopause Reset Timeline

A well-structured timeline is the backbone of your menopause reset plan. It helps you organize your goals and strategies effectively. Here's how to create a menopause reset timeline:

- Start with the End in Mind: Visualize where you want to be at the end of your menopause reset journey. This could be a state of reduced symptoms, improved overall well-being, and greater confidence.
- Identify Short-Term and Long-Term Goals: Divide your menopause reset journey into short-term and long-term goals. Short-term goals may focus on immediate symptom relief, while long-term goals could revolve

around maintaining your well-being post-menopause.

- Assign Timeframes: For each goal, allocate a specific timeframe. Short-term goals may have deadlines ranging from a few weeks to a few months, while long-term goals could span several months to a year or more.
- Sequential Order: Arrange your goals and strategies in a logical, sequential order. For instance, if you're starting an exercise routine, make it a short-term goal before progressing to more advanced fitness objectives

## Finding Support and Accountability

Embarking on a menopause reset journey can be challenging, but you don't have to go it alone. Finding support and accountability can significantly enhance your chances of success.

Consider these sources of support:
- Healthcare Professionals: Consult with a healthcare provider who specializes in menopause or hormonal health. They can provide expert guidance, recommend treatments or therapies, and monitor your progress.

- 
- Support Groups: Joining a menopause support group or online community can connect you with others experiencing similar challenges. Sharing your experiences and receiving advice from peers can be empowering.
- Friends and Family: Share your goals and progress with trusted friends and family members. They can offer emotional support and encouragement.
- Accountability Partners: Partner with a friend or family member who can hold you accountable for your goals. Regular check-ins and shared goals can keep you motivated.
- Health and Wellness Coaches: Consider working with a menopause or wellness coach who can provide personalized guidance and motivation throughout your journey.

Keep in mind that requesting help is a sign of strength, not weakness. It can make your menopause reset more manageable, enjoyable, and ultimately successful. Don't hesitate to lean on your support network when needed, and celebrate your progress together as you work toward feeling like your younger self again.

# Chapter 10: Maintaining Your Progress

Maintaining the progress you've made during your menopause reset is a crucial aspect of managing this life transition effectively. Menopause is not a one-time event; it's a journey that can span several years. Here are some essential strategies for maintaining your progress:

1..Consistency is Key: Continue to follow the lifestyle changes and treatment plans that have worked for you. Consistency in your diet, exercise, and other practices is vital for long-term success.

2. Check-Ins: Make regular appointments with your healthcare practitioner. These appointments will help you assess your hormone levels, monitor your progress, and make any necessary adjustments to your treatment plan.

3. Lifestyle Integration: As you progress, integrate the changes you've made into your daily life. Make them part of your routine rather than temporary fixes. This includes sticking to a healthy diet, exercise regimen, and stress management techniques.

4. Ongoing Education: Stay informed about menopause and related health issues. Knowledge is power, and staying up-to-date will help you make informed decisions about your health.

5. Listen to Your Body: Pay attention to your body's signals and symptoms. If new issues arise or existing symptoms worsen, don't ignore them. Consult with your healthcare provider to address any changes promptly.

6. Self-Care: Prioritize self-care as an ongoing practice. Menopause is a time when self-compassion and self-nurturing are essential. Make time for relaxation, hobbies, and activities that bring you joy.

**Tracking Your Symptoms**

Tracking your menopause symptoms is a vital part of managing your health during this phase of life. Here's why it's vital, and how to do it properly:

1..Understanding Your Body: Symptom tracking helps you understand how menopause affects your body. It can reveal patterns and triggers for specific symptoms, which can inform your treatment plan.

2. Effective Communication: When you visit your healthcare provider, having a detailed symptom log can facilitate more productive discussions. You can provide specific information about your experiences, making it easier to tailor treatments.

3. Identifying Trends: Over time, tracking allows you to identify trends in your symptoms. For example, you may notice that certain symptoms worsen during stressful periods or improve with particular lifestyle changes.

4. Choosing the Right Interventions: With a clear symptom record, you and your healthcare provider can make informed decisions about which

interventions are most effective for your unique situation.

5. Utilizing Technology: Consider using apps or digital tools to track your symptoms conveniently. These tools often provide helpful charts and graphs that can simplify the tracking process.

## Adjusting Your Plan as Needed

Flexibility is key when it comes to managing menopause. Here's how to adjust your plan effectively:

1..Regular Reassessment: Plan for periodic assessments with your healthcare provider to evaluate your progress and adjust your treatment plan as necessary. Menopause is a changing process, and your needs may shift.

2. Open Communication: Maintain open and honest communication with your healthcare staff. If you experience side effects or feel that your current treatments aren't effective, discuss these concerns promptly.

3. Lifestyle Modifications: Be willing to make adjustments to your lifestyle plan. If certain exercises or dietary choices aren't working for you, consult a specialist or nutritionist to modify your approach.

4. Medication and Hormone Therapy: If you're on hormone replacement therapy or medication, your healthcare provider may need to adjust dosages or switch to different options based on your response and any new health considerations.

5. Holistic Approaches: Consider incorporating holistic approaches such as acupuncture, mindfulness, or herbal remedies into your plan if you believe they may offer benefits.

## Celebrating Your Successes

Celebrating your successes, no matter how small is an important part of maintaining motivation and emotional well-being during your menopause reset:

1..Set Milestones: Establish achievable milestones along your journey. When you reach them, take a moment to acknowledge and celebrate your accomplishments.

2. Self-Reflection: Periodically reflect on how far you've come and the improvements you've experienced. They can offer emotional support and comprehension.

3. Reward Yourself: When you complete a key objective, treat yourself to something unique. It could be a spa day, a new book, or a night out with friends.

4. Share Your Achievements: Share your successes with friends or support groups. Celebrating together can strengthen your sense of community and provide additional motivation.

5. Positive Self-Talk: Practice positive self-talk and self-encouragement. Remind yourself of your resilience and the progress you've made.

## Finding Support and Accountability

Support and accountability are crucial elements of a successful menopause reset. Here's how to find and utilize them effectively:

1..Lean on Loved Ones: Share your menopause journey with friends and family. They can provide emotional support and understanding.

2. Join Support Groups: Consider joining local or online menopause support groups. These communities can offer advice, empathy, and a sense of belonging.

3. Professional Guidance: Seek out healthcare providers, nutritionists, fitness trainers, and mental health professionals who specialize in menopause. They can offer expert guidance and accountability.

4. Accountability Partners: Find an accountability partner with similar goals. Having someone to check in with and share your progress can help you stay motivated.

5. Online Resources: Explore reputable websites, forums, and social media groups dedicated to menopause. Just be cautious of misinformation and always consult professionals for personalized advice.

In conclusion, successfully navigating the menopause reset involves maintaining progress, tracking symptoms, adjusting your plan, celebrating achievements, and seeking support and accountability. By actively managing your menopause journey, you can improve your overall well-being and embrace this phase of life with confidence and vitality.

# Chapter 11: Life After Menopause

Menopause, the biological milestone marking the end of a woman's reproductive years, is a transformative phase in a woman's life. But what comes next, in the post-menopause phase, can be equally fascinating and empowering. Embracing life after menopause means acknowledging that your journey is far from over; it's a chance to rediscover and redefine yourself in ways you may not have expected.

**Embracing the Post-Menopause Phase**
Self-Discovery and Empowerment: Post-menopause is a time for self-discovery and self-empowerment. With the cessation of menstrual cycles and hormonal fluctuations, many women find a renewed sense of freedom. They can focus on personal growth, pursuing long-delayed dreams, and embracing new challenges.

1..Physical and Emotional Freedom: The end of menopause-related symptoms, such as hot flashes and mood swings, often brings a sense of liberation. You can fully engage in life without being hindered by these symptoms. This newfound freedom can lead to a more positive and optimistic outlook.

2. Reconnecting with Your Body: Post-menopause is an opportunity to reconnect with your body in a different way. Regular exercise, a balanced diet, and mindfulness practices can help you maintain overall health and well-being. Many women report feeling more in tune with their bodies during this phase.

3. Reinventing Relationships: Your post-menopausal years can also be a time to reinvent your relationships. With a deeper understanding of yourself and your desires, you may find that your connections with loved ones become richer and more fulfilling.

**Sexual Health and Intimacy**
1..Redefined Sexual Expression: Menopause doesn't signal the end of sexual activity—it marks a shift. Some women experience increased sexual desire and satisfaction after menopause due to the relief

from concerns about pregnancy. Others may face challenges like vaginal dryness or reduced libido, but there are solutions available, from lubricants to hormone therapy.

2. Open Communication: Open and honest communication with your partner is crucial during this phase. Discuss your desires, concerns, and expectations to maintain a healthy and satisfying intimate life. Many couples find that post-menopausal intimacy can be more meaningful and fulfilling.

3. Regular Check-Ups: Regular gynecological check-ups remain essential to monitor your sexual and reproductive health, even after menopause. Your healthcare provider can address any concerns, recommend treatments, and ensure you continue to enjoy a satisfying sex life.

## Maintaining Long-Term Wellness

1..Healthy Aging: Post-menopause is a time to focus on healthy aging. This includes maintaining a well-balanced diet rich in calcium and vitamin D to support bone health, engaging in regular exercise to preserve muscle mass and cardiovascular health, and practicing stress reduction techniques to support mental well-being.

2. Bone Health: Osteoporosis risk increases after menopause due to declining estrogen levels. Discuss bone density testing and appropriate interventions with your healthcare provider to safeguard your bone health.

3. Heart Health: Cardiovascular health is vital in the post-menopausal phase. Regular check-ups, cholesterol monitoring, and a heart-healthy lifestyle can help prevent heart disease, which becomes a more significant concern as estrogen levels drop.

4. Mental and Emotional Well-Being: Post-menopause can bring about emotional changes, such as increased self-confidence, but it can also be a time when some women experience mood swings or depression. Seek support and professional guidance if needed to maintain emotional well-being.
In summary, life after menopause is a unique and exciting phase of a woman's journey. Embracing it involves self-discovery, self-empowerment, and a focus on overall well-being. It's a time to nurture your physical and emotional health, maintain

satisfying relationships, and pursue your passions with renewed vigor. By understanding and embracing the post-menopause phase, you can look forward to a future filled with opportunities, growth, and fulfillment.

# Conclusion

**Embracing Your Younger Self Again**

In the final chapter of "The Menopause Reset," we arrive at a pivotal moment in your menopause journey—embracing your younger self again. While it may sound paradoxical, menopause offers a unique opportunity for rediscovery and renewal, a chance to reconnect with the essence of who you once were while celebrating the wisdom and resilience you've acquired along the way.

**Reflecting on Your Menopause Journey**

To truly embrace your younger self again, it's essential to reflect on the incredible journey you've undertaken. Menopause is not just about the physical changes or the sometimes challenging symptoms; it's a profound transformation that affects your mind, body, and spirit. Take a moment to acknowledge the strength it took to navigate this transition. You've weathered the storms of hormonal fluctuations, the often bewildering emotional shifts, and the physical transformations that come with this phase of life. You've emerged on the other side, transformed and renewed.

As you reflect on your menopause journey, consider the valuable lessons you've learned along the way. Menopause is a teacher, offering insights into your body, your resilience, and your capacity for adaptation. The challenges you've faced have made you stronger and more self-aware. Take pride in your ability to persevere and grow through this transformative experience

# Homemade Recipes for Menopause Reset

Recipes tailored for menopause can play a significant role in managing symptoms and promoting overall health and well-being during this life stage. Menopause brings hormonal changes that can lead to various physical and emotional challenges, such as hot flashes, mood swings, weight gain, and bone health concerns. A well-balanced diet with specific ingredients and nutrients can help alleviate some of these issues. Let's explore some unique and nutritious recipes designed to support women during menopause.

**1. Hormone-Balancing Smoothie:**
**Ingredients:**
1 cup unsweetened almond milk
1/2 cup Greek yogurt (rich in probiotics)
1/2 banana (potassium-rich)
1 tablespoon flax seeds (omega-3 fatty acids)
1/4 cup mixed berries (antioxidants)

1 teaspoon maca powder (supports hormonal balance)

1/2 teaspoon turmeric (anti-inflammatory)

Honey or maple syrup (optional, for sweetness)

**Instructions:**

Blend all the ingredients until smooth.

Adjust sweetness to your liking with honey or maple syrup.

Enjoy this nutritious smoothie as a breakfast or snack to help regulate hormones and reduce mood swings.

## 2. Bone-Boosting Quinoa Salad:

**Ingredients:**

1 cup cooked quinoa (calcium-rich)

1 cup cooked broccoli (vitamin K for bone health)

1/2 cup chickpeas (good source of protein)

1/4 cup diced red bell pepper (rich in vitamin C)

2 tablespoons chopped fresh parsley (contains boron for bone health)

2 tablespoons lemon juice

1 tablespoon olive oil

Salt and pepper to taste

**Instructions:**

In a large bowl, combine quinoa, broccoli, chickpeas, red bell pepper, and parsley.

In a small bowl, whisk together lemon juice, olive oil, salt, and pepper.

Drizzle the dressing on the salad and toss for it to combine.

Serve as a nutritious lunch or dinner option to support bone health during menopause.

### 3. Relaxing Herbal Tea Blend:

**Ingredients:**

1 teaspoon dried chamomile flowers (calming)

1 teaspoon dried lavender buds (stress relief)

1 teaspoon dried sage leaves (hot flash relief)

1 teaspoon dried red clover blossoms (hormonal balance)

8-10 ounces boiling water

Honey (optional, for sweetness)

**Instructions**:

Combine the dried herbs in a teapot or infuser.

Pour boiling water over the herbs and steep for 5-7 minutes.

Strain the tea into a cup, add honey if desired, and enjoy this soothing herbal blend in the evening to promote relaxation and relieve menopausal symptoms.

**4. Calcium-Packed Green Smoothie:**
**Ingredients:**
1 cup kale (excellent source of calcium)
1/2 cup unsweetened coconut milk (rich in calcium)
1/2 ripe avocado (healthy fats)
1/2 cup mango chunks (vitamin D for calcium absorption)
1 tablespoon chia seeds (calcium and omega-3s)
1/2 teaspoon vanilla extract
Honey or maple syrup (optional, for sweetness)
**Instructions**:
Blend kale, coconut milk, avocado, mango, chia seeds, and vanilla extract until smooth.
Adjust sweetness with honey or maple syrup if needed.
This smoothie provides a calcium boost essential for bone health, which can be crucial during menopause.

**5. Mood-Stabilizing Salmon with Quinoa:**
**Ingredients:**
2 salmon fillets (rich in omega-3 fatty acids)

1 cup of cooked quinoa ( that is high in protein and fiber)

1 cup steamed asparagus (folate for mood support)

1 tablespoon olive oil

1 lemon, thinly sliced

Fresh dill for garnish

Salt and pepper to taste

**Instructions**:

Preheat your oven to 375°F (190°C).

Season salmon fillets with salt and pepper and place them on a baking sheet.

Lay lemon slices over the salmon, drizzle with olive oil and sprinkle with fresh dill.

Bake it for about 15-20 minutes.

Serve the salmon over a bed of quinoa and steamed asparagus for a mood-stabilizing dinner that's rich in omega-3s and essential nutrients.

**6. Menopause-Friendly Snack:**

**Ingredients:**

1 small apple, sliced (fiber for digestive health)

2 tablespoons almond butter (healthy fats)

A sprinkle of cinnamon (anti-inflammatory)

A pinch of ground flaxseed (omega-3s)

**Instructions**:

Slice the apple and arrange it on a plate.

Drizzle almond butter over the apple slices.

Sprinkle cinnamon and ground flaxseed on top.

Enjoy this nutritious and satisfying snack that provides fiber, healthy fats, and anti-inflammatory benefits, which can help manage menopause symptoms and cravings.

**7. Anti-Inflammatory Turmeric Soup:**

**Ingredients:**

1 tablespoon olive oil

1 onion, chopped

2 carrots, chopped

2 celery stalks, chopped

1 teaspoon ground turmeric (anti-inflammatory)

1 teaspoon ground ginger (digestive support)

4 cups vegetable broth

1 cup red lentils (protein and fiber)

Salt and pepper to taste

Fresh cilantro for garnish

**Instructions**:

Preheat olive oil in a large pot with medium heat.

Add chopped onion, carrots, and celery. Sauté until the vegetables are tender.

Stir in turmeric and ginger.

Pour in the vegetable broth and add red lentils.
Bring to a boil, then reduce heat and simmer for
about 20 minutes.
Season with salt and pepper.
Serve with fresh cilantro for added flavor and anti-
inflammatory benefits.

## 8. Berry Blast Menopause Smoothie:

**Ingredients:**

1 cup mixed berries (antioxidants)

1/2 cup spinach (iron and folate)

1/2 cup unsweetened almond milk (low in calories)

1 tablespoon hemp seeds (omega-3 fatty acids)

1/2 teaspoon ground flaxseed (fiber)

A touch of honey or agave syrup (optional, for
sweetness)

**Instructions**:

Combine the mixed berries, spinach, almond milk,
hemp seeds, and flaxseed in a blender.

Blend until smooth, adding honey or agave syrup if
desired.

This refreshing smoothie is packed with antioxidants
and nutrients to combat oxidative stress and support
overall health during menopause.

## 9. Collagen-Boosting Vegetable Stir-Fry:

**Ingredients:**

1 cup broccoli florets (vitamin C for collagen production)

1 cup bell peppers, thinly sliced (rich in antioxidants)

1 cup snap peas (collagen-boosting vitamin K)

1 cup tofu or tempeh (plant-based protein)

2 cloves garlic, minced

2 tablespoons low-sodium soy sauce or tamari

1 tablespoon sesame oil

Sesame seeds for garnish

Cooked brown rice (optional, as a base)

**Instructions:**

Preheat sesame oil in a large skillet with medium or high heat.

Add garlic and sauté for 1-2 minutes.

Add broccoli, bell peppers, snap peas, and tofu or tempeh.

Stir-fry for about 5-7 minutes until vegetables are tender and tofu is slightly crispy.

Drizzle it with soy sauce or tamari and toss it to coat.

Serve over cooked brown rice, if desired, and garnish with sesame seeds.

This collagen-boosting stir-fry is not only delicious but also supports skin health during menopause.

**10. Menopause Comfort Herbal Tea:**
**Ingredients:**
1 teaspoon dried sage leaves (hot flash relief)
1 teaspoon dried licorice root (hormone balance)
1 teaspoon dried black cohosh root (menopausal symptom relief)
8-10 ounces boiling water
A touch of honey or lemon (optional, for flavor)
**Instructions:**
Combine the dried herbs in a teapot or infuser.
Pour boiling water over the herbs and steep for 5-7 minutes.
Add honey or lemon to give flavor if you want and to your desire.
Sip on this herbal tea to help alleviate hot flashes and other menopausal discomforts.
These recipes focus on ingredients that can help address specific menopausal symptoms, such as hot flashes, mood swings, bone health, and collagen production. Incorporating these recipes into your diet can contribute to a healthier and more comfortable menopausal experience. As with any dietary changes, it's essential to consult with a

healthcare professional or nutritionist to ensure they align with your individual needs and health goals. A well-balanced diet combined with holistic approaches can enhance your overall quality of life during this phase of womanhood.

# 7 Days Meal Plan for Menopause

A well-balanced and nutritious meal plan is essential for managing menopause symptoms and promoting overall health and well-being during this life transition. Here's an extensive and unique 7-day meal plan designed to help you navigate menopause with vitality and comfort. Please note that individual dietary needs and preferences may vary, so consider consulting a healthcare professional or nutritionist for personalized advice.

**Day 1: Hormone-Balancing Start**
**Breakfast**:
Greek yogurt parfait with fruit and honey drizzle
Chia seeds for added fiber and omega-3 fatty acids
**Lunch**:
Grilled chicken breast salad with mixed greens, avocado, and balsamic vinaigrette
A small serving of quinoa or brown rice for sustained energy
**Snack**:
Sliced cucumbers and carrot sticks with hummus
Dinner:

Baked salmon with lemon and herbs
Steamed broccoli and asparagus
Sweet potatoes on the side for complex carbs

**Day 2: Plant-Powered Day**
**Breakfast:**
Spinach and mushroom omelette with feta cheese
A slice of whole-grain toast
**Lunch**:
Lentil and vegetable soup
Whole-grain crackers
**Snack**:
Mixed nuts and a piece of fruit
**Dinner**:
Stir-fried tofu with colorful bell peppers and broccoli
Quinoa or brown rice as a base

**Day 3: Anti-Inflammatory Delights**
**Breakfast:**
Overnight oats with almond milk, flaxseeds, and sliced bananas
A sprinkle of cinnamon for flavor
**Lunch**:
Kale and Brussels sprout salad with walnuts and cranberries

A light olive oil and lemon dressing
**Snack**:
Greek yogurt with a dash of turmeric and honey
**Dinner**
Grilled shrimp with garlic and ginger
Sautéed spinach and quinoa

## Day 4: Omega-3 Richness
**Breakfast:**
Smoked salmon with cream cheese on whole-grain bread
Tomatoes and red onion, sliced
**Lunch**:
Salad of quinoa and black beans with cilantro-lime dressing
**Snack**: sliced avocado on top
**Dinner**: a handful of blueberries and walnuts
Cod baked in a lemon-dill sauce
Steamed asparagus with wild rice on the side

## Day 5: Mood Enhancing Flavors
**Breakfast**:
Waffles made with whole grains, almond butter, and sliced strawberries
**Lunch**:

Wrapped roasted chicken and vegetables with tahini drizzling

A garnish of mixed greens

**Dinner:** Celery sticks with peanut butter

Stir-fry beef and broccoli with ginger and garlic

Low-carb options include brown rice or cauliflower rice.  potatoes for complex carbohydrates

**Day 6: Bone Health Focus**

**Breakfast:**

Spinach and feta stuffed whole-grain crepes

A sprinkle of sesame seeds

**Lunch**:

Butternut squash soup with a side of whole-grain bread

**Snack**:

Low-fat cottage cheese with pineapple

**Dinner**:

Baked chicken thighs with rosemary and lemon

Roasted Brussels sprouts and quinoa

**Day 7: Hydration and Detox**

**Breakfast:**

Green smoothie with spinach, kale, banana, and almond milk

A scoop of protein powder for added energy

**Lunch**:
Tomato and cucumber salad with red onion and basil
A light balsamic vinaigrette
**Snack**:
Sliced apple with a drizzle of honey
**Dinner**:
Grilled vegetable platter with a tahini-yogurt dip
A small serving of couscous or bulgur wheat

Remember to stay hydrated throughout the week by drinking plenty of water and herbal teas. Adjust portion sizes according to your individual needs and activity level. This meal plan emphasizes whole foods, fiber, healthy fats, lean protein, and a variety of fruits and vegetables, which can contribute to hormone balance, manage weight, and alleviate common menopausal symptoms. Additionally, be mindful of your unique dietary preferences and any specific allergies or sensitivities you may have when following this meal plan.

# Appendix

**Recommend Websites:**

**North American Menopause Society (NAMS) - [www.menopause.org]:** NAMS is a reputable organization dedicated to advancing the understanding of menopause and improving women's health during this life stage. Their website offers a wealth of evidence-based information, resources, and expert advice.

**Mayo Clinic - [www.mayoclinic.org]:** Mayo Clinic's website provides reliable information on menopause, its symptoms, treatment options, and practical tips for managing this phase of life.

**WebMD Menopause Center - [www.webmd.com/menopause]:** WebMD offers an extensive online resource center specifically focused on menopause, including articles, videos, expert interviews, and user forums for community support.

**The Menopause Exchange - [www.menopause-exchange.co.uk]:** This UK-based website offers a range of articles, newsletters, and resources related to menopause, catering to an international audience.

**HealthyWomen - Menopause - [www.healthywomen.org/menopause]:** HealthyWomen provides valuable insights into menopause, covering a wide range of topics from symptom management to lifestyle adjustments.

**Support Groups:**
**Menopause Matters Forum - [www.menopausematters.co.uk/forum]:** An online community where women can share their menopause experiences, seek advice, and provide support to one another in a safe and understanding environment.

**Red Hot Mamas - [www.redhotmamas.org]:** Red Hot Mama
s offers in-person and virtual support groups, educational programs, and resources for women navigating menopause.

**Smart Patients - Menopause Community - [www.smartpatients.com/communities/menopaus e]:** An online forum that connects women going through menopause, allowing them to discuss their experiences, ask questions, and find support from a global community.

**Local Meetup Groups**: Check platforms like Meetup.com for local menopause support groups in your area. These gatherings provide an opportunity to connect with women in your community who are experiencing similar challenges.

**Facebook Menopause Support Groups:** Numerous Facebook groups are dedicated to menopause discussions, offering a virtual space for women to share their stories, ask questions, and receive support.

These recommended resources are designed to complement your menopause journey. Remember that every woman's experience of menopause is unique, so exploring different sources and seeking support can help you tailor your approach to this transformative phase and ultimately regain a sense of balance and well-being.

www.ingramcontent.com/pod-product-compliance
Lightning Source LLC
Chambersburg PA
CBHW070822260726

48660CB00005B/1953